BOASTING
IN
MY WEAKNESS

BOASTING
IN
MY WEAKNESS

ALYSE CLARK

To God: I am truly nothing without you. My desire is to walk in the purpose for which you created me, daily.

To my husband: Thank you for loving me, supporting me, and encouraging me to live out my dreams. You are my biggest cheerleader and my best friend.

To my children: I thank God for you. You inspire me to live, and I hope you know that I believe you will soar much farther than I can even think of going.

To my parents and family members: Your support has given me the confidence to aspire to greatness and not allow societal norms to put limits on me. I am so thankful to be a part of something so much bigger than me.

To the memories of Elder Sarah A. Nettles and Minister Mattie A. Austin: Eld Nettles taught me to embrace who I am. She was not afraid to do things that were different and in so doing, she accomplished what others thought could not be done. Min. Austin inspired me from afar. She taught me that just living your best life can be an inspiration to others. I am blessed to have known them both.

CONTENTS

"NORMAL"

Throughout this book, I use the word *normal*. When I think of the word normal, I am referring to what I have accepted as the standard of practice. In my case, it is the standard of practice in my day to day and how my life looks as I try to navigate it. As I travel on this journey, I realize that my standard of practice or my normal has not been healthy. I have been driven by this internal need to accomplish as many tasks as I can. The problem with this is that many times, the number of tasks that I take on is not reasonable. There is a trend in the work world to get more with less. Some call that efficiency. How can I get more work from people and not spend more money? Work with a smaller staff and ask them to not only do more work but also require them to keep up with the increasing needs of the industry or organization. Then you hire the type of people who have a "get 'er done" mentality. These people will work themselves to death, literally.

Throughout my career, I have watched this play out in my own life. I've never been afraid of working hard. I've taken it as a challenge and have enjoyed the accomplishment, especially when others benefit. When I was younger, it began with my eagerness to try new things and me jumping at every opportunity to learn and grow. The first time I thought about the load I carried occurred when I gave up one of my advisor positions. The principal had to find two people to take my place. I was still young and naïve. I didn't realize what I should have learned from that. When it spoke to my inability to live a life of balance, I thought it spoke to my abilities. People wanted me on their team because they knew I would work. Over time, I would let this define me. I was proud of the fact that I could work hard and get things done. I rarely stopped to think about the unreasonable expectations that I allowed others to put on me and that I put upon myself. By the end of this story, it became my norm to do the work of two people. In my later years, I didn't think it was fair, and finally I asked God to show me what I was doing wrong. I wondered why I kept getting the short end of the stick. The Lord gave me my answer. One evening, I was scrolling through social media, and I happened upon a discussion that was being conducted by two of my former students. They were talking about "Finding Peace in the Chaos." As I listened to their conversation, God spoke to me. I was having a tough time finding the time to do what I needed to do. I had made a commitment to myself that home would be home and work would be work. This became a need because I felt like I was not giving enough time to my family. Over the years, I had become used to working long hours and bringing hours of work home. This was normal for me. I didn't understand those in my profession who didn't bring hours of work home. This was the norm in our profession. Most of the people with whom I worked agreed that this was the expectation. Not only did I bring hours of work home, but I also worked all day without breaks. I ate lunch while I worked. Sometimes I didn't eat lunch until after 2 p.m. Sometimes I didn't eat at all. I would give my job nine non-stop hours during the day and then bring hours of work home. As I struggled with my chronic conditions, I found I couldn't even think well enough in the evenings to continue working for hours. I was exhausted and could barely make it past dinner time. As my children were getting older, they wanted more time with me, and I was exhausted. My husband was understanding, but he needed me too.

As I struggled to find balance, I also struggled with the guilt of not giving my family the time that they deserved. During the pandemic, I worked from home like many others. This worked out great for my job as I began spending twelve hours a day in my office working. I can't tell you how many times my husband would bring my dinner to me in my office as I completed one more meeting or one more project. Even when I would stop and eat dinner with the family, I would go back to work after dinner. My children would come into my office in the evenings and sit around on their tablets as I worked because they wanted to spend time with me. I knew something had to change. This could not be my life. It wasn't fair to my family. I didn't think it was fair to me. It wasn't what God wanted for me.

This story is my journey to freedom. Jesus told the Pharisees that the truth would make them free. As I learn to walk in the truth of what God has said about me, I find a freedom that I never realized was possible. God wants us to live a life of freedom so we can be who He wants us to be. Sometimes, one of the most difficult things for us to do is to face our truth. We worry about what people will say. This is because we often live a life of comparison. We understand that living a life of comparison means that we are more concerned with what people think than with what God says.

God has not called us to pursue a normal existence. I learned this lesson as I pursued normality in my own life. God will allow disruptions in our lives to get us where He wants us to be. This is my truth. As I learn to walk in the truth about who God says I am, I can truly boast in my weakness.

Chapter One

OCTOBER 29TH

I remember this night clearly. It was a Sunday night about 9 p.m., and I was lying in bed. I felt a sense of accomplishment because I had finished the laundry and I was in bed on time. I was watching television, and I felt good. While I was lying there still and relaxed, I remember thinking that my heart was beating faster than normal. It seemed like something that I couldn't ignore, so I turned to my husband to ask him to chek and see if he thought there was anything unusual about the speed of my heartbeat. I turned my head toward him and tried to speak to him. When I opened my mouth, there was a sound, but I could not say his name. The sound I heard was more of a grunt. I thought, *Am I crazy? Did that just happen?* I was determined in my mind to say his name again. No words came out when I looked at him and opened my mouth. I could make noise, but no words, and I also realized that I couldn't move my left arm or leg. My husband had been listening to something on his phone, so I had to keep making noise until I got his attention. He turned to me, and I kept trying to communicate with him. He realized I couldn't talk, and I could barely move. Tears rolled down my face, and he tried to comfort me. I saw the look of concern as he reached across my torso to grab the phone. I don't think I will ever forget him saying to the 911 operator, "I think my wife is having a stroke." *How could I be having a stroke?* I thought, *I don't smoke. I don't drink. My blood pressure is low, and I have lost weight.* It was unreal. Even though I lost the ability to speak, and my movement was severely limited, I was aware of everything that was happening. Somehow, I could communicate with my husband so he could put on some more clothes as we waited for the ambulance to arrive. My two youngest daughters were sleeping. My oldest daughter sat in the living room with me. I looked at her, and even though I didn't know what was happening to me, I didn't want her to be afraid. I tried to tell her to take care of her sisters. My husband had called my parents, and they were on their way to the house.

The paramedics got me into the ambulance and rushed me to the emergency room. When I got there, so many people helped me. The room was large, and it was unlike any ER experience I had before. Soon a screen came toward me, and there was a doctor on the screen asking me questions. By then, I was regaining the ability to speak, and I could tell her what happened. She suspected that I may have had a TIA or mini stroke. She explained that after a TIA, people usually regain the ability to speak and move. They admitted me for further testing. I was confused. I couldn't imagine what caused this. The doctor ordered an MRI and an EEG and tried to further assess my situation. I remember one resident was rude to me during this time. Blood tests showed that my B12 was low, and he assumed I had been neglectful and brought this upon myself. He was wrong.

They discharged me a day later, and I was to see my doctor for a follow-up appointment. When I left the hospital, I was walking and talking fine. The doctor said it was a suspected TIA, and I left confused but happy that I was better. The morning of my follow-up appointment, I told my husband that I would be fine driving myself to the doctor's office. It was very close to our house, and I felt fine. As I began getting ready for the appointment, I was going over what happened (talking to myself) so that I could give my doctor all the information she needed. As I went through the story in my bedroom, I noticed that my speech was slowing down. I called my husband and asked him if I sounded normal as I spoke to him. He said no and informed me he would drive me to the doctor's office.

By the time I got to my appointment, I knew that something was wrong. When I tried to sign the papers at the office, I could barely write my name. I tried to stay calm because I really didn't want to alarm my husband. It was too late for that. He knew something was wrong and decided that he was going back into the exam room with me. I would like to take a moment here to express how important it is to be or have your own advocate for health care. The nurse did not realize that I was losing the ability to speak and moved me right in front of her. She took my blood pressure and temperature as usual. By the time she left the room, I could barely speak. I had all the words in my head, but most of them wouldn't come out. I could only express myself using one or two words per sentence. My husband went to get the doctor. When she saw the state I was in, she had someone call 911. She assessed my situation. I would come to understand that this was how doctors assessed patients to see if they had a stroke. As I tried to answer the questions from the EMT, my doctor informed him that this was not how I normally spoke. I realized that he just thought I was a mentally disabled patient. Once again, I was rushed to the emergency room in an ambulance. This time, when they admitted me, they placed me in a stroke unit and began testing me again. I had a 24-hour EEG so they could see what was going on in my brain when I had these "attacks." They discharged me after four days in the hospital. The EEG didn't show any abnormalities. They thought maybe it was hypoglycemia since my blood sugar was low when the ambulance brought me in. They assumed that this might have caused my problem. So, I left with a blood glucose meter and instructions to eat more snacks. As a side note, I'm never mad about snacks.

After all of this, I still did not know why this happened to me, and I realized the doctors didn't know either. It seemed like this issue came out of thin air. When I went to my follow-up appointment with my doctor, she mentioned she had another patient with similar issues, and it turned out to be a migraine. She referred me to a neurologist who, after assessing my situation, determined I was having migraine with aura.

Now, one thing you can know about me is that I research every-thing. I love to learn and be knowledgeable. By now, I had researched every symptom and test that I had experienced. I looked up migraines with aura, and I really saw nothing that truly matched my situation. In fact, I wasn't even experiencing headaches. One thing the neurologist let me know was that there was no cure for migraines. I really didn't understand what I was going through, and I had nothing to warn me about what the future would bring. This first stage of my illness would last about twelve days between hospital and doctor visits. After seeing the neurologist, we scheduled a follow-up visit, and I returned to my normal routine.

Everything went back to normal until one day in July. I decided it was time for me to clean out my little girls' closets. It was a big job, and I felt a sense of accomplishment when I finished until I experienced another attack. This time, armed with the information the neurologist gave me, I realized I had overdone it, and that seemed to have caused the attack. In the future, I would have to be more careful about physical work. I thought I was figuring this thing out. I still didn't know why it was happening, but at least I was learning enough to control it, or so I thought.

That next fall, a year after the first attack, more attacks greeted me. This time, they were more frequent. One time, I was in the car on the way home from church. By the time we got in the driveway, I couldn't talk and I couldn't walk. It was horrible. I didn't want my kids to be afraid. My husband had them go into the house first. My oldest was a teenager. She kept the little girls busy in the living room while my husband got me out of the car and into the house. Until this point, my attacks usually happened first thing in the morning. My husband would get the kids ready and take them to school. They didn't have to see what was happening to me. It's hard to explain things to your children when you don't know what is happening yourself.

After a few days, I was better. I made it to the Saturday before Thanksgiving. My Saturday routine involved an early morning trip to the grocery store. I liked to go early when few people were there. I returned home, put my groceries away, and began prepping for Sunday dinner. While I was working in the kitchen, I noticed I was limping. I hadn't hurt myself, and I wasn't in any pain, but it seemed like I had developed a limp. Once again, I wondered if I was losing my mind. At nap time, I put the kids down for a nap. No one was home but me and the little girls. While they were napping, I walked across the living room floor to see if I really had a limp. I couldn't understand how I was limping, and I hadn't hurt my leg. How do you just develop a limp when you've never had one before? When my husband got home, I showed him what was happening. We decided I should rest, and I did. When I got up the next morning, it was worse. My husband took me to the emergency room. As a result of this emergency room visit, they admitted me for more tests. More MRIs. Even though I did not enjoy being in the hospital, I must admit that this time I could overcome one of my fears. When I was pregnant with one of my daughters, they needed to do an MRI to find the source of the blood clots that traveled to my lungs as I was thirty-two weeks pregnant (this is another testimony). They could not complete the test because I found out at that moment that I was claustrophobic. After that, they gave me a sedative if they needed to conduct an MRI. This time, they forgot to give me the sedative. I had waited twenty-four hours to be tested, and I didn't want to wait another day. When I got to the room where they conduct the test, I prayed, asked them to cover my face with a towel, took a deep breath, and prayed my way through that MRI. I haven't had a problem with them since. Praise God! The MRI came back normal. They discharged me with a cane, a prescription for physical therapy, and an appointment with my neurologist.

I made it out of the hospital in time for Thanksgiving. After the holiday, I began physical therapy. For the next four weeks, life was rough. I had this limp from nowhere, and I was experiencing "migraine attacks" three to four times during the week. It was hard on me. It was hard on my family. I was struggling to do simple things for myself. My husband would get up with the kids, and my mother would come to the house to make sure I would be okay while he was gone. Sometimes unusual symptoms would become part of the attacks, and during those times, I would end up in the emergency room. Once they gave me a migraine cocktail in the ER. This is a cocktail of drugs that they give patients suffering from migraines. I have had two migraine cocktails in my life, and I never want one again. They administered intravenously a migraine cocktail. This allows the drugs to enter your system quickly. The first effect is extreme anxiety as your body goes into extreme relaxation. I know that relaxation sounds like a good thing, except it's involuntary. Losing control over my body was not a good feeling. By the end, the Benadryl kicks in, and you go to sleep. It was a nightmare.

I went to physical therapy two times each week. They worked with me to teach me how to walk with a cane and to exercise my leg, hoping that the muscle memory would kick in at some point. I tried to be as normal as possible. I struggled so much in the beginning that I had to use a wheelchair if we went into the stores. Even though the wheelchair made it easier for me to get around the stores, I was embarrassed to have to use this type of support. Older people would help me get things from the shelves when I couldn't reach them. It was a lot to deal with, and I still didn't know what this was or why it was happening.

Besides physical therapy, I was to undergo more tests. This included another MRI, as well as nerve and muscle tests. I hoped that this would give me the information I needed. I wanted to put a name to this problem, and that meant more to me than fixing it.

We made it through the holiday season, and on January 17, we sat with the neurologist as he gave us the results. He told me that all my tests came back normal and said that this (the limp) might be an emotional problem. I didn't understand what he was saying. I said, "Are you saying this isn't real?" He assured me that the limp was real. He suggested that somehow stress was causing my brain to not communicate with my leg. Walking with a cane helped me coordinate my leg while I suffered with this condition. I must admit that it devastated me. I had a real problem but no solution. The doctor prescribed medication that he said might help, and I needed to take the pills every day. I started taking the medicine and continued using my cane. I wouldn't have another attack until June, but I would be on the cane for the next six months. Then one day in May, my leg started working again. I didn't know what happened, but I was happy to be off of the cane. By then, it had been one year and seven months since October 29. I had more symptoms and no diagnosis, no real understanding of why this was happening, and it was so unpredictable. I tried to watch my level of stress. Maybe that would help.

Chapter Two

THE IMPORTANCE OF FAMILY

It was very frustrating to be suffering from sickness and have very few answers about why it was happening, what it was, and whether there was a cure. I think one of the hardest things about dealing with my condition was watching the reaction of my loved ones, especially my husband.

My husband was not totally surprised about dealing with me and sickness. When we were dating, I was recovering from bilateral pulmonary embolisms, also known as blood clots, in both lungs. The interesting thing was that prior to my first incident with pulmonary embolisms, I had not had to deal with sickness. Prior to that, the only sickness I had was chicken pox as a seventeen-year-old. I've never even had the flu, praise God. So, imagine my surprise when, a week after surgery, I couldn't catch my breath after minimal activity. I had been staying with my parents as I recovered from surgery. The day before my follow-up visit with the surgeon, I was struggling to catch my breath after walking a short distance. When I called the nurse, she told me to rest and if things got worse, I should go to the emergency room. I must admit that I was horrible at self-care. By the time it was time for bed, I knew something was wrong. I should have gone to the emergency room then, but I never imagined that my condition was life-threatening. That night, as I got ready to go to bed, I remember praying a prayer that differed from any I had prayed before.

I told God that no matter what happened, He was still the King of Kings to me. I can honestly say that God kept me through the night. I had been diagnosed with sleep apnea and used a BiPAP machine while I slept. This machine facilitated breathing in and breathing out as I slept. I would come to realize that this machine would be a provision that night. By the time I got up in the morning, I didn't have the energy to get myself ready for my doctor's appointment. It had been a week since I had surgery, and it was time for my follow-up appointment with my surgeon.

I thought I was just weak because I was on a clear liquid diet after the surgery. A few days before, the visiting nurse had said that I could have apple juice mixed with water to help boost my energy. My mom had left a bottle of apple juice on the kitchen counter for me, and as I stood there trying to catch my breath so I could try to open it, I realized I couldn't breathe. A wave of anxiety swept over me as I struggled to breathe. I cried out, and my mother came out of her room to see what was wrong. I told her I couldn't breathe. Her response was all too familiar. She is a prayer warrior, so she did what she does best. I can always count on my mom to pray. I never had an experience like this before, and she thought I was having a panic attack. I didn't know any better, so I thought the same. The next few hours were unlike any I had ever experienced before. By the time we got to the doctor's office, I told my dad that I didn't have the strength to walk from the parking lot to the doors of the office. My dad let me out at the door, and I waited in a wheelchair at the entrance of the building as older and elderly people walked by me. My father pushed me into the building and onto the elevator. When we got to the doctor's office, I was determined to walk back to the examination room. Every movement took all my energy. I struggled to keep up with the nurse as she led me to the room where they would take my weight and blood pressure. The blood pressure machine was not working. We had to walk all the way back to the last room. I sat down and asked the nurse to give me a minute while I tried to catch my breath. She took my blood pressure and escorted me to the room where I would meet with the doctor and nurse practitioner.

When my surgeon saw me and I told him what was happening, he sent me to the hospital as a precaution. His office was next to the hospital, so my dad pushed me over in a wheelchair. They did a CT scan and told me I had blood clots in my lungs. I didn't even realize how serious this was. I remember sitting in admissions in the hospital, telling my dad "At least it's not life-threatening" as I continued to struggle to catch my breath. It wasn't until later, when I had been admitted and subjected to tests, that I would find out why I was struggling to breathe. By then, my mother was there. She had been waiting at home for hours. I had left her house going to a follow-up doctor's appointment, and my father had to tell her I had been admitted to the hospital.

I remember the pulmonary specialist explaining to us I had blood clots in my right thigh that broke loose, went through my heart, and settled in both lungs. I remember him telling us he felt encouraged because "if this was going to kill you, it would have happened yesterday." It was at that moment that I understood the severity of my situation. I spent seven days in the hospital and, at my mother's insistence, I went back to my parents' home once I was discharged. After two days, they let me go home. I lived alone, and my parents just wanted to make sure that I could take care of myself.

I went through all of this before I started dating my husband. My parents and my brother were there for me through this time, and it made me look at life a little differently. I was grateful that God spared my life. My condition was quite serious, and I was blessed to be alive. I thought about life and how I was spending my time. I had dreams and plans and I would often tell myself that I would pursue my passions after I retired. This experience made me realize I might not even live to see retirement. And then what? I changed my focus. I felt like I had been given a gift, and I didn't want to waste my life not living it the way God intended.

While I was working through this experience, I didn't understand how it was affecting my family. Until then, I had been pretty independent. I would call my parents daily just to let them know I was safe. I was used to traveling by myself, and I was responsible. After the blood clots, I was more intentional about traveling with my brother, so my parents knew I wouldn't be by myself if something happened. I didn't realize the impact this experience would have on my life. My immune system was compromised because of the blood clots, and I became susceptible to more illnesses. My body had been through trauma, and I didn't have normal strength. As I climbed the mountain of recovery, I would experience setbacks that seemed to knock me back a few yards. One thing I remember is how my father would call me and encourage me through these times. I am not really someone who will readily share when things aren't going well. I just suffer through the best way I can. My father would always call at the right time with the right word. I have always known him to be a man who follows God. He always had a timely word for me.

As I mentioned before, I had been independent, and I liked that. This experience made me more vulnerable. I was going to work to gain back my independence, but I realized it was better for me to get help. I am so thankful that my family was there for me.

It was shortly after this that I started talking to my husband. I had seen him at church conventions, but I never talked to him. While I was going through this, he was going through a transition in his own life. Since we lived in different states, we spent most of our time talking on the phone. Early in our conversations, he expressed to me that God had told him I was to be his wife. I told him God had not informed me of this. He encouraged me to pray, and I did. In all honesty, I wasn't looking for marriage. I had been single for many years, and I had accepted my singleness and planned to live my best life as a single woman dedicated to God. In my prayers, God let me know I could trust this man with my heart.

I was glad that we had a long-distance relationship. We could spend most of our time talking and getting to know each other on the phone. As our relationship grew, my husband knew he was going to marry me and was working on a plan to take care of me since he knew about what I had suffered. He pursued me, knowing that I was sick, and committed to taking care of me even when neither he nor I knew what that would mean for our future. As we got closer to our wedding day, my mother would tell me that she and my father were no longer worried about me once he came into the picture because they knew he would be there when I needed him.

My husband has been there to hold my hand through this journey. I've said before that I didn't understand what was happening, but I realized that it was even more terrifying for him. As a man, he took his job of protecting me very seriously. He was suffering because he couldn't protect me from this illness. I try to remember that when I become impatient with him because I feel like he is being overprotective. My father has told me that you can do anything if you are committed to it. This experience has helped me to understand true commitment in a marriage. Our commitment to each other is greater than any illness.

I am so thankful for the family that God has given me. I hoped to always be there for them. I felt like I had so much to give to my family, and I was happy to do so. As I have struggled through this part of my life, they have consistently been there for me. One of my struggles in life has been to accept help from others. I loved the fact that I could help someone, but I never really thought about the time when I needed help. I've learned that part of humility is acknowledging the times when you need help. We always need God's help, but He often uses people to provide that help. The ministry of family is God's creation. My family has been there for me throughout this journey, and they have been my motivation to keep fighting for me.

Chapter Three

I'M STILL IN HERE

A day after my first hospitalization for symptoms that would become known as hemiplegic migraine, I went to the doctor for a follow-up. This is normally what one does after you have been in the hospital. The follow-up is so your doctor can work with you to develop a care plan. While in the office, as I mentioned in an earlier chapter, I had another episode. I didn't know what was happening to me. I looked at my husband, and he looked concerned. With what little language I could use, I said, "I'm still smart." I remember that moment so well because, little by little, I was losing control of my body. I couldn't control a pen to write my name. The words in my head were not coming out of my mouth. I felt like I was going crazy. In my head, everything was normal, but I couldn't get my body to cooperate. I could see and hear what was happening to me, and I didn't look or sound like me.

Ever since I can remember, I've had an excellent memory. As a child, I could memorize long speeches for church. As I grew older, I relied on my memory more and more. I have even memorized my debit card number. My memory has truly been an asset in my life. I remember once thinking, *What will I do if my memory fails me?* As we get older, our ability to remember things decreases. I thought I had many years to worry about that. Thinking and problem-solving are things that I really enjoy. I even had a supervisor tell me, as I was navigating through this sickness, that he wasn't worried about me performing physical duties, as long as I could still use my brain. I knew I was blessed to have success in areas where I had to think, and I enjoyed it. Once I had a diagnosis and read and learned more about this disorder, I realized it was all in my brain. I wondered if I would lose cognitive ability as well. I found that metal fatigue was a genuine issue, and when I became overwhelmed, I couldn't think straight. My attention span decreased. Sometimes it was hard to focus. Once again, I couldn't do what I normally did. Multitasking became more difficult for me. I struggled to remember how to play songs on the piano that I had played for years. I wondered if I really was still smart. Fear set in, and I kept this secret to myself. I had to work, and I felt like my choices were limited. I requested information and a retirement application after I investigated disability retirement. I remember, while in my conference, the person telling me that if I retired on disability, that I could not teach again. I was struggling, but those words rang in my head. Was I ready to give up teaching? Was I ready to give up my passion?

Over the years, I have learned that teaching is a gift that God has given me. It amazed people how I could reach my students, but they didn't realize that it amazed me as well. I loved watching the light bulb come on for students. Ideas would come to my mind, and I would try them. I was so excited when these ideas worked. As I progressed in my career, I found the same joy in watching the light bulb come on for adult learners and even in lessons that I taught in church. I realized that teaching is my passion, and

I was not ready to give it up. That stopped me from pursuing disability retirement. I wasn't sure what I was going to do, but it wasn't time to give up. I knew God had more for me to do.

I've learned throughout this journey that my battle is not my disorder. If God allowed me to experience this, it would be good for me. I had to get to the place where my faith in God allowed me to see this. Initially, I saw these disorders as barriers in my life. I saw the limitations, but I now know that they serve a greater purpose.

One movie that I really like is *The Wiz*. In that story, Dorothy is on a journey to get the help she needs to get home. The journey takes her to a place in which she realizes that she always had everything she needed to get home within herself. I can relate to this story. My focus on the limitations associated with having disorders has taken me in a circle. I have felt trapped by the idea of being disabled. If I accepted these disorders, then I could not be me, or so I thought. Sometimes I am having an episode and I am fully aware of everything that is happening to and around me, yet I am no longer a participant. I want to move my left arm, but I can't. I want to speak, but I can't. The words and actions are so clear in my mind, but I cannot manifest them. When I'm having a rough day and fatigue has a grip on me, I want to push through so people don't notice. I don't want them to ask me what's wrong because I really don't know. Even though I sleep all night, I am still tired, and I don't always know why. I find it takes days to gain normal strength, but I don't have the days, and I feel guilty if I take them. I'm not normal anymore, and that's all I want to be. The beginning of this journey was to "still be me." I wanted to be the "me" that every-one, including me, expected. I had set a standard for myself that I thought was good, and this new normal did not allow me to be the person whom I had become comfortable being. There were areas in which I wanted to be better. I had other goals for myself. As I journeyed through life, I learned to put those goals to the side until I retired. After I had the blood clots, I realized I might not live to retire. Then what? If I died, what did I have that I had done for myself? I am a person who believes only what you do for Christ will last. If I was being honest, my life had become more about what I did for people than what I did for Christ. I wasn't doing wrong, willfully sinning, or mistreating others. In fact, I often put my well-being to the side to do what I felt others wanted me to do. I didn't want to let anyone down. Even when I was sick and in the hospital, I worked and did things for other people. In some sad way, it made me feel good. I felt like I was still living up to this high standard I set for myself. I would not let these disorders stop me from living. This is what I told myself. The more I pushed to be normal, the more I suffered. My body was telling me that I couldn't keep functioning like this, and I was trying to fight reality. Then one day, I was honest with myself. I told myself, "I can't do this any-more." By this time, I had been tested for diabetes only to find out that I was suffering from low blood sugar. The specialist told me that I needed to change my diet so I didn't have the blood sugar spikes. We were working like crazy in the middle of a pandemic. I didn't eat regularly. I wasn't get-ting good sleep, and I started having episodes on a weekly basis. I knew

36

that I was in a bad place. I saw my neurologist, and he told me that the blood sugar spikes, along with missing meals and sleep, were like slapping my brain back and forth. So now, in addition to having this disorder, I was causing my own problems. I had to make some major changes.

I took some time to focus on myself. During that process, the Spirit led me to embrace my conditions. Until that time, I felt imprisoned by my conditions. I was trapped, and I felt like it was because I had a clotting disorder and hemiplegic migraine. Initially, I believed they were things I needed to overcome. When I embraced them, things changed for me. In *The Wiz*, a storm brought Dorothy to a place where she could face things she was missing, and she overcame by realizing that she had these things all along. I realized it took the storm of sickness to put me on a journey of finding what I already had. I need to confront the lies by which I was living. God has so much more for me, and I had become satisfied with less than what God wanted for me. There is a genuine danger in aligning your goals with the world's standards. This is how we miss out on God's purpose for us. I had dreams, and I had allowed my career path to detour me. After my career was done, I felt like I could pursue my dreams. I thought it was my duty to excel in my career, and after a while, my focus was off. The storm of sickness shook the foundation on which I was building my life. I love God, and I was doing what I knew to do for Him. Again, I wasn't willfully sinning. That's why I could go to Him when I was sick. I could lean on Him, knowing that He would keep me. What I didn't realize was that He was going to reveal some things to me about myself. Once He showed me, it was my choice to make changes. I realized that my intelligence, my gifts, didn't matter if I did not use them for God's plan. I could be at the top of my career, making a great salary, and none of that mattered to God if it wasn't where He wanted me to be. I could be the best choir director, musician, preacher, or church member by the pastor's standard, and it wouldn't matter to God if I didn't fulfill my calling.

The "me" that felt trapped by my disorders wasn't the "me" that God was calling me to be. Until that point, I was the best me I could be, but God was calling me to be greater. He let me know that everything He put in me, every experience He allowed me to have, was to push me to greater in Him. I was satisfied with where I was in life. I had a good job. Life was comfortable. So, when things got uncomfortable, I fought to get back to that same level of comfort. In my mind, the choice was: I could be who I was or be less than who I was. I hadn't considered that I could be better. I was so focused on my abilities that I forgot to look to God. Living with limitations brought on by these disorders is what I saw. I looked at myself based on how I thought the world would see me.

It was difficult to embrace my new normal. I still have many challenges, but the challenges are mine, so I can win. The first step is learning not to let what others say or think define or deter you. Sometimes the greatest battle is what we *think* others are saying. Know that this is a trick of the enemy. Remember, he is a liar. He brings thoughts to trap us in a state of "not doing." That's all he wants to do. If he can stop us from following God's plan for our lives, he is satisfied.

Chapter Four

SECRETS AND LOSS

People who know me will say that I am a private person. To me, this means that I keep a low profile. I rarely make special efforts to hide information from others. I just don't make special efforts to share a lot of personal information with people. I'm pretty transparent about my life. When asked, I will share my experiences, especially my mistakes, hoping they will help someone else. I've been blessed to accomplish many things in life. Sometimes I think it's good for people to understand that we all have challenges to overcome.

With my disorders, I'm not ashamed. I spent most of the beginning of the journey just trying to find out what was happening to me and why. There were times during hospital stays in which I wondered if I could even return to work. I struggled to maintain the standard I had for myself in my professional life. I kept pushing, trying to keep some sense of normalcy amid this new chaos. Everyone was concerned about me, and that made me even more uncomfortable. I didn't want to be disabled. I didn't want people to think that I couldn't do the things I normally did at home, work, or even church.

I've learned that people often fear what they don't understand. I wanted people to know that I still had my life. People who cared about me didn't want me to "be sick." I didn't either, but as long as I still have life,

I'm going to live it. I knew I wasn't ready to give up, and I didn't want to be sitting in a corner, so I decided I wouldn't tell people about my conditions if I didn't have to.

I had been on my job for many years and had many experiences and accomplishments over the years. My conditions were quite challenging. One of the hardest parts of the struggle was that the doctors were still conducting tests to rule out conditions so they could come up with a diagnosis for me. Here I was with a cane, and I couldn't tell people why. I never want people to feel sorry for me, but I had to think about what I would do if this was to be my future. What if things got worse? What if I had to use a walker or a wheelchair? None of the doctors were telling me I couldn't work. Honestly, many of them were unsure about my condition as well. I thought that my best bet would be to live as normal of a life as possible. I wasn't ready to give up my career or my church work, so I would try to figure out how to manage in this new normal.

My strategy was to keep my conditions to myself. I would only tell people if I felt like they really needed to know. I didn't want people to pity me, and I didn't want them to limit me from doing things I wanted to do. My conditions were challenging me, but I had a strong will to live. I didn't want to be put in a corner. Eventually, I learned that people's reaction to my situation was more about their comfort level than mine.

As life moved forward, I needed to find a new job. We had moved to a new city, and I needed to work. I was blessed with an excellent position. My husband would ask me if I told them about my disorder, and

I would always tell him "Not yet." I decided I would only tell them if I absolutely had to. I didn't want people to judge me before they could see what I could accomplish on the job.

I would eventually find out that keeping my secret would complicate things. Chronic illness had taken many things from me, and I didn't realize it. I thought I could find the right medicine or change my working habits and then I would be okay. I thought I could keep my secret until I managed my disorders. When I first began seeing a neurologist, he told me that there was no cure for my condition. My first hematologist told me I would take the medication he prescribed for the rest of my life. They were both telling me something that I didn't understand. My conditions were chronic. I would often talk about getting used to a new normal, and I would eventually find out that my definition of normal would have to change. Over time, I realized that loss would accompany my conditions. With loss comes grief.

I've read some things about grief. Usually, when we think about grief, we speak of losing someone like a loved one. Clinicians have defined the distinct stages of grief that eventually take us to accepting the loss. I learned that these stages of grief are also present with chronic illness. My journey is taking me to a place where I have to accept that there are things that will never be the same for me. Things in my life that I counted on are now gone. These statements are not rooted in hopelessness. I root them in acceptance. I didn't want to accept what I saw as the limitations of my illnesses. I didn't want to be sick. I didn't want to lose anything. I wanted to get back to being the same as I was before. That was denial. If I could push through like everything was fine, I would be okay. The problem with this theory was that the more I pushed through, the more I suffered. My symptoms got worse. I could barely function, and it was affecting me and my family. As I kept trying to function as if nothing was really wrong with me, I felt guilty as I had no energy to give to my family. Most of our time together was spent with them taking care of me. When I spent all of my energy at work, I suffered for it at home. I felt guilty about taking sick days when I could barely get out of bed. When I took a sick day, I felt like I had to keep up with the work even though I was bedridden. I would show them I could crank out my work, even from my hospital bed. I felt guilty about missing church services and other church obligations. Again, I would be in the ER or the hospital or bedridden, but somehow, I felt like I needed to push through. I thought I could win this way.

Eventually, I would understand that I couldn't do things like I used to do them. I would deal with anger and sadness. When that reality sank in, I understood the loss associated with chronic illness. There were so many things that I wanted to do in my life, and I couldn't see how I could accomplish these things, considering what I had lost. I also felt like I was letting everyone down. I just didn't have the strength and energy to carry on, and I didn't want to tell people about what I was going through. I didn't understand this part of grief and how important it is to process it in a healthy way. I learned it is okay to mourn loss. It's natural, and it's not a permanent state. Once I accepted the fact that I couldn't do things the way I once did them, I started making changes. These changes were necessary and would help me move toward living a better life. These changes didn't cure me of the illness, but they would help give me a better outlook on living with them.

I am tired most of the time. Chronic fatigue goes along with my conditions. One of my prescribed medications causes fatigue as well. Sometimes people say, "You look tired." Well, I feel tired, so I'm glad I'm not crazy. I understand I will be tired, so I've learned to be careful about how I spend my physical and mental energy. I have no more energy to spend on keeping secrets about my condition. I can no longer spend energy acting like I am one hundred percent when I am not. I will spend no more energy trying to prove that I can outwork everyone else with less energy and strength. This is who I am. If it pleases God for me to live with these conditions, then I am happy to do so.

Sometimes I have felt so down. The feeling was not really a result of my illnesses. It resulted from me looking at the long list of things that I would struggle to accomplish because I lacked the energy, and I knew that if I pushed through and did them anyway, I would suffer an attack and the additional days I would need to recover. It is in the acceptance of this reality that I have gained one of my greatest victories. I am a person who suffers from chronic illness/disease. This reality is something I embrace. I have realized that the things that I have lost are no longer needed in my life journey. There was a time when I needed to learn lessons those experiences brought me. Now the lessons learned have become values in my life. This is much like our experience with reading in school. When we learn to read in the primary grades, there is an emphasis on spelling tests and vocabulary tests. These are tools we need to develop our reading fluency. As we grow older, schools focus on reading comprehension. The end goal is that we can read words accurately, understand what we are reading, and then use what we have read to apply to other things. By the time you get to high school, if you are still focusing on spelling words, something has gone wrong in your reading journey.

Life is the same way. I don't define my effectiveness by the number of tasks I complete. The quality of the tasks matters. The quality of the experience is more important than the number of experiences. It's not the number of interactions, it's the quality of the interactions. It's not the number of times I can show up, it's how I show up. I needed to lose everything I have lost in this season. My mentality had to change. I needed to grow into the next stage of life, and I couldn't go into that stage with the habits of the last one. The experiences that led to achievement in my last season were great, but those experiences will not lead to success in my next one. That can be hard for us to understand as human beings because we love to exist in a comfort zone. So, God allows us to go through different challenges. If we are totally committed to Him and to living our lives according to His purpose, those challenges will not break us. These challenges have forced me to seek God for guidance. God has shown me through this experience that it was time for me to shift.

As I move through the last stages of grief for the things that I once counted as lost, I am thankful and hopeful. I have learned a great deal from these experiences, and I am now empowered with more knowledge. Knowledge with experience will bring about wisdom. Life has taught me that wisdom allows you to move through life more strategically. People call that learning to work smarter. The Bible says that God calls on the young because they are strong and the old because they know the way. When I was younger, I placed most of my life's value on my strengths. As I grow into maturity, I am learning to appreciate using wisdom. I really struggled with what I lost, but I realized that it was time for me to transition into the next season. That doesn't mean that what I had wasn't good. It just means that it's time for me to change. Change is difficult for us as human beings. I am thankful for God's grace and mercy. In a time when I needed to change, He allowed me to lose things that were blocking my progression. This is how I learned to take pleasure in my weakness.

Chapter Five

FEELING CHEATED

". . . You do not belong to yourself, for God bought you with a high price. So you must honor God with your body." (1 Cor 6:19–20 NLT)

One of the greatest battles is between the flesh and the spirit. This is something we often hear and come to learn in our walk with Christ. What this means is that we have a constant struggle with what we can see and feel in our natural experience as we try to walk in the spiritual reality to which God has called us. The only way we can walk in spiritual reality is through the Holy Spirit by faith. The battle is that while we have real, natural life experiences, we must base our hope and actions on what God says. This does not mean that I act like what I am experiencing is not real. It means that I keep going, pursuing God's will for me even when I can't see how I can do it. We achieve this reality through experience with God as we go through life's temptations.

I have to be transparent here. It seems like these conditions came out of nowhere. I didn't see warning signs, and while I am truly thankful I am still here, I have struggled with understanding why. It seems like I waited my turn for so many things in my life and tried my best to do it the right way. These conditions have taken my physical strength. Everything is so much harder now. I've worked to manage my conditions, and just when it seems like I have it together, something else comes to complicate matters. If I'm being truly honest, I have felt cheated as I am going through this part of the journey. I am grateful for life, and as much as that is true, I have struggled to figure out what that life is supposed to look like now. In my mind, there are so many things that I have wanted to do, and my body just won't cooperate. I have spent so much time trying to prove that I can still do what I've always done, and I have suffered for it. As tired as I am, I have wanted to give up, but something doesn't let me. At times, I have struggled to figure out if it is hope or stubbornness. I've often said that I didn't want people to feel sorry for me, but the actual battle is for me not to feel sorry for myself. As a Christian, I thought I could not feel this way. If I'm trusting God, then how can I feel cheated? If His will is what's best for me, why can't I glory in this tribulation?

During this experience, I have had some "real moments" with God. I have cried to Him in ways I didn't even know I would. I'm learning that our flesh is going to have actual feelings, and the way we work through them is to take everything to God. The Scripture lets us know Jesus can be touched by the feeling of our infirmities and that he was tempted just like we are, but He didn't sin. I don't feel ashamed of how I feel. I just have to make sure that my actions don't reflect the reality of my feelings. My actions must reflect the reality of my faith in God to be all that He says he is. It is natural to feel cheated when you feel like so much is being taken from you. We have to get an understanding like Job, who realized that the Lord "giveth" and the Lord "taketh." This means that instead of my disease taking, God took it. How much time do we spend trying to keep something that God no longer wants us to have? When God takes something, He is letting us know that it no longer has value in our spiritual journey. God wants us to trust Him totally.

Building a trusting relationship can take time. I am learning that I show my trust in God by trusting His judgment. As I have grown older, I have had many experiences and have developed my own understanding about how things should go in my life. According to societal standards, I can say that I have shown pretty good judgment. When things happen in this life, we rely on our own judgment and experience. This is an extremely limited way of thinking. God has all knowledge of everything. There is nothing He does that is not intentional. During many trials, I have quoted Romans 8:28: "And we know God causes everything to work together for the good of those who love God and are called according to his purpose for them" (NLT). I must admit that I had to learn what that Scripture really meant. There is a good that we understand from our perspective, and then there is a good from God's perspective. The natural loss that I have experienced didn't feel good to me. It didn't look good. I had to understand that I can't see everything that God sees, so I couldn't see the benefits. Since we cannot see like God can, we must trust that He is leading us on the path that will be most beneficial. To do this, we must learn to walk by faith in His word. Even though I was losing what I knew, I had to first believe that God knew what was going on and was still in control of my life. That meant that I had to be thankful for every part of this journey. I had to believe that God allowed these things to happen to me because it was what was best for me. I had to believe that there were things that God no longer wanted me to have, so He took them so I could be in a better position with Him. We often talk about what the devil stole. We want it all back, but what if God took these things as part of my maturation process?

I looked to God for strength when I couldn't rely on my strength anymore. When I could no longer trust my brain, I prayed to God to give me understanding. When I could no longer be sure that my legs would work correctly, I turned to God to guide and strengthen me. I found that this new normal for me was so uncertain that I struggled to make decisions about work. This has been one of the most difficult things for me to conquer. I have confidence in my ability to do the job, but it is a struggle for me to keep up with the day-to-day demands of the job. In the past, I was always up for the challenge. I enjoyed handling difficult situations, and I loved finding solutions to situations that seemed too difficult to handle. This new normal would bring me to a place where I struggled to keep up with all my responsibilities. Most of the time, I lived with unrealistic expectations for myself. I spent well beyond the daily work time to make sure that I finished tasks at a high level. I took on any challenge that was thrown in my direction and volunteered for some that weren't. This wasn't just at work. It felt good to me that I could be counted on to do whatever someone asked me to do. Many times, this meant staying up late into the night and sacrificing my rest and health. This became my reputation, and I had been proud of it. Once I had to deal with these conditions, I could no longer keep up with my own standards. I didn't know how to approach tasks anymore, so I felt cheated. This is the other reason we must learn to trust God. I've learned that you can't trust your feelings. I felt cheated because I could no longer carry out unrealistic expectations that were killing me. God was leading me down a path that would allow me to live a life I didn't realize was possible.

When we moved to a new city, I got a new job, and one of the supervisors had worked with me early in my career. After I got the job, she expressed confidence in my ability to do the job well. She said, "She's a workaholic." Though she meant that as a compliment, those words would haunt me. I used to be a workaholic, but I was no longer proud of that. I knew that being a workaholic was not healthy, and it was cheating me of a good life. It was an addiction, and the payoff was just as detrimental as a narcotic. When you have addictive behaviors, you live life through an unclear lens. Your judgment about what is reasonable or even normal is poor.

An addict is one exhibiting a compulsive, chronic, physiological, or psychological need for a habit-forming substance, behavior, or activity (*merriam-webster.com*). Usually, when we think of an addict, we think of someone being addicted to drugs, food, or even work. The addiction is more about the feeling we get from the substance or behavior. One can gain a chemical dependency on drugs, but it was the feeling one got from being high that led them to taking drugs. When one develops a food addiction, it is the feeling of comfort associated with eating that causes the person to continue to go to the food. It's the same thing with the addiction to working. For me, it was the feeling of accomplishment or achievement, especially when it seemed like the task was nearly impossible. At first glance, that doesn't seem like a terrible thing. What's wrong with feeling good about a job done well? The problem occurs when that feeling drives your actions. When that feeling becomes most important, it can take you to a self-destructive place. There's nothing wrong with pursuing excellence, but we have to be careful when we allow it to consume us in such a way that we pursue it at all costs. This is why God calls for us to enjoy things in moderation. We must have balance in our lives and an understanding that our focus has to be on pleasing God, not on natural accomplishments.

Our feelings will always betray us. We may never feel a sense of accomplishment when we are working to please God. This is a faith walk. For my daughter's birthday, we decided to go to a restaurant for dinner. As we entered the building, I saw a sign that asked patrons to use the door to the left. The sign was posted at eye level and was printed in bold black letters on a white piece of paper. We had about a thirty-minute wait before we could be seated. As we sat, I was able to observe many people coming into the restaurant. Several people opened the door that had the sign on it, and I was able to see why they asked people not to use that door. It amazed me that even though the sign was visible, people opened the door anyway. I don't think people were ignoring the sign. I believe that people were used to walking by faith in using doors. When people see a door, they automatically try to open it. They have faith in a system that says if a business has a door and it's during normal business hours, the door should open when you pull the handle. The owners of the restaurant understood the system as well, so they put a sign on the door to try to get people to change their behavior. Every person who opened that door had the same issue. They didn't read the sign.

In our spiritual walk, we must have faith in God. God's system also requires that we watch and pray. As human beings, we get into patterns and habits of behavior. We spend time perfecting good behaviors with the expectation that we will be successful. When our good behaviors take us to a place where we no longer feel successful, we struggle. Walking by faith in God is not perfecting good behavior. It is about learning the voice of God and following Him without knowing where He is going to take us. As a human being, the feeling of uncertainty is real. This is why we have to learn to trust God completely. Following God will take you to places that challenge your senses. The ability to continue to move forward will not be based on how you feel. I move forward knowing that I am following the directions that God has given me. Jeremiah 29:11 says, "For I know the thoughts that I think toward you, says the Lord, thoughts of peace and not of evil, to give you a future and a hope." In this scripture, God is telling Jeremiah that He knows the purpose to which He called him. It is the same for me. God knows how He wants to use me in this life. The things that I go through in this life are designed to get me to that purpose. I cannot allow my feelings to deter my progress.

Chapter Six

QUESTIONED FAITH

The healing power of God is something in which I honestly believe. I believe God can heal me. I have uterine fibroids. During my first pregnancy, I discovered this. During my fourth month of pregnancy, one fibroid degenerated. For me, the pain of a degenerating fibroid was worse than labor pains. The hospital gave me morphine, and I spent some days on bed rest. This was one experience I had during my first pregnancy. I would add that the pregnancy ended early, as I had pulmonary embolisms, severe anemia, and other issues. When I found out that I was pregnant with my second child, I believed I was healed of these issues. I prayed and believed that when they did the ultrasound, there would be no fibroids. When I went in for my first ultrasound, I expected to see a miracle. I expected the fibroids to be gone. I knew it would amaze the doctors, and I would have a testimony to tell. The day came, and when they did the ultrasound, the fibroids were still there. I knew I believed God would heal me, but clearly it was not His will.

As I experienced the episodes that go with hemiplegic migraine, I prayed for healing. The ministers laid hands on me. I searched the Scriptures about asking God for things in faith. I believed God would heal me one day. This is something I believed with everything that I had in me. Now let me tell you what I know about God. He is sovereign, which means He can do whatever He wants. So, if there was a problem in this situation, it was me. I would hear testimonies about how people believed God, and He healed them. I would hear messages about asking and seeking, and I was trying my best to do this in my situation. During this process, I learned some things about God that I didn't know previously.

Just because we believe in God does not mean that He is going to do what we want or how we want it. I have always known that we could ask God for anything, according to His will, and He would grant it. Surely it was God's will to heal me, right? I was struggling. I couldn't do things the way I used to do them. I was even missing church services. This can't be God's will for me, can it? As I progressed through this journey, God gave me a Scripture, 2 Corinthians 12:9. That scripture is His answer to Paul, who is suffering with infirmity in his own flesh. Like me, Paul sought the Lord multiple times for deliverance. God's response to him was that this infirmity had a purpose in Paul's spiritual walk, and He comforts Paul by letting him know that the grace of God is sufficient for this situation. He also lets him know that in our weakness, God's strength works best. With this assurance, Paul responds with an attitude change about his infirmity. This scripture has become my battle cry.

The faith that I need to access in this situation is not about God's ability to heal me from these physical infirmities. It is about my ability to trust that God has a purpose for allowing these illnesses and disorders to become a part of my existence here on earth and still believing that I can do all things through Christ who strengthens me. I have understood that

God has a purpose in everything He does, and His focus is His Kingdom. As we learn to give our lives to God, we will find the need for a mind shift (Rom 12:1–2).

Once I went to a funeral for a small child who had a severe cognitive disability. He died at about four years of age. It was incredibly sad. During the service, I heard people talk about how positive the child was in life. Several people expressed memories of joy as they reminisced about encounters with this child. Society does not associate joy with the potential of a child with severe disabilities. In fact, doctors will give parents options to end a pregnancy if they believe the child will be born with a severe disability. Some would say that the child won't have a quality of life even if they live beyond the expected age. I sat at the funeral encouraged because I realized this child had served his purpose in four short years, and when his assignment was over, God took him. What I learned from this is that God values things we don't. Often, we human beings value the wrong things. This can lead us to put our faith in the wrong things as well. This means that we are often asking God for the wrong things. I wanted to be healed from these physical disorders and discomforts so I could do what I had been doing the way I had been doing them. After a while, I had to make a decision. When I realized God was not going to heal me physically, I had to decide if I was going to give up on life or live an abundant life. In all honesty, I wanted to quit. I was so tired. Physically, I struggle to do what was once so normal to me. Deep in my heart, I knew that quitting wasn't an option, and I came to realize, after years of struggle, that this was an opportunity for me. This was an opportunity for me to trust God in a way that I had never trusted Him before. I was so focused on limitations and what I could no longer do. Many mornings, I cried out to God as I struggled to get out of bed, "Lord, please help me!" I felt like I knew what needed to be done each day, but I didn't have the strength, and I felt like I didn't have any choices. This sounds like a familiar line from a familiar gospel song, "My back was against the wall." I felt like I was losing so much. There was one fact that I held onto even in the times in which I struggled the most. I knew God was faithful, and I knew that even though I didn't understand what was happening to me and why, I could trust that He knew what was best for me. That doesn't mean I didn't feel bad. It doesn't mean days were easy. It means that I never felt hard toward God. It means that even on the worst of days, I still looked toward God for comfort. I still remembered that I owed God praise, even when I didn't feel like it. I still had hope.

Again, I learned that having faith in God doesn't mean that He is going to do everything I want Him to do. It means that I can trust that He has ordered my life, and if He is allowing me to go through these things, then it is good for me. The key has become for me to change my attitude and thinking about what God allows in my life. That means I have to adopt His standard and abandon my own. I had aligned my standard with societal standards (the world). What good can come of sickness and weakness? I never wanted to be seen as sickly. I did not want to be seen as weak, but according to God's word, it is in my weakness that His strength can work perfectly. This let me know I don't have to rely on my strength. I can rely on God. Whatever God wants me to do, I can do because of His strength, not mine. This is even more exciting because even on my best day, my strength cannot match God's. So, I have discovered through this sickness, this weakness, that I was always living a life of limitations. I was focused on my strength, my knowledge, and my ability. When all those things failed, I had to learn to rely on God for things that were once normal to me. I would pray to ask God to give me strength to work a normal work-day. I would pray to ask God to give me strength to cook dinner and do my children's hair. My testimony matched the song that says, "I can't even walk without you holding my hand." As I became more intentional about trusting God for everything, my mind shifted. I started letting go of the desire to excel in the areas that I had traditionally excelled in and embraced the idea of moving in a direction that God was leading me into. These were dreams I believe God has given me, but I couldn't see in my mind how I could accomplish them. As I learned to trust God in my new normal, I realized that I no longer had to rely on my ability. There are no limits in God. It took this experience to get me here. God wanted to heal me spiritually. He wanted to deliver me from my own thoughts that were limiting my vision. He wanted to take the hurt of disappointment that had resulted in fear.

This part of the journey is quite interesting. I learned to embrace this new normal, but I still found it difficult to walk in it. Once my father told me that if you start walking by faith, you have to keep walking by faith. As simple as that sounds, it's something to think about. I accepted the fact that I had these conditions, and I believe God was still with me. I now had to trust that God would carry me through, no matter how I felt. Walking through this situation by faith and not by sight was my new goal. Many days, I feel bad, yet I still need to go to work. I don't see how I can keep working, and I don't see how I can afford to stop working. I wake up each morning and thank God for life. Then I ask Him to help me through the day. I believe if I live my life in obedience to Him, He will make a way for me each day. I've gotten to the place where my focus is more on walking in my God-given purpose by obeying Him daily. This is how I continue my faith walk. I have learned that walking by faith doesn't mean that I won't feel bad. Contentment with God is not an emotion. It's a spiritual reality that goes beyond our feelings. It's a state of mind. My emotions are largely based on the circumstances that I may be experiencing. I may feel sad and overwhelmed because I am extremely tired and have a lengthy list of tasks that I need to accomplish. In this situation, I don't feel good. In those times, I cannot complete the tasks like I think I should. I may not have the capacity to get them done at all. Operating in a state of contentment with God helps me to prioritize my life. As long as I do what God says first, then I rely on Him to direct me on how to accomplish other things. The Scripture tells us to seek kingdom things first and not to worry about the cares of this world, knowing that God will take care of those things as He cares for us. When we can walk in this Word by faith, we will find the peace that only God gives. For me, the feeling of being overwhelmed comes from the reality of having so much to do and limited ability within myself to accomplish things. Often, even in my healthier days, these tasks would be overwhelming. In those days, I would have worked until I completed every task. I would not have rested until I completed them. The problem is that they are never truly completed. The feeling of accomplishment is fleeting because once you have climbed one mountain, you can see the mountains that await you. The more you do, the more you must accomplish. It seems to never end. I have now learned to seek contentment with God. The Scripture tells us that Godliness with contentment is great gain or wealth. It lets me know that true value is in finding contentment with walking in God's way. That same Scripture goes on to let us know that we came into this world with nothing, and we will leave this world with nothing, so we have to learn to be content with our basic needs being met. God often provides beyond our basic needs. It is our desire to have excess that leads us down a path to destruction. The system of this world encourages us to seek this excess under the misnomer of living a "good life." We will run ourselves ragged to have "things" and never genuinely enjoy them. It's a trap and a distraction. When we truly learn to walk by faith, we trust God to supply what we need, knowing that He provides according to His purpose for us. His provision is not just economic. He supplies strength and knowledge according to His purpose as well. So, when I find my natural strength lessened, my faith tells me that I still have more than enough to accomplish God's purpose in my life. The battle is not fighting to get more strength. The battle is accepting what God allowed to happen in my life, knowing that He is in control.

Chapter Seven

THE BLESSING OF WEAKNESS

Sometimes I experience ataxia as a symptom of hemiplegic migraine. Ataxia is the lack of muscle control or coordination in voluntary movements. For me, this means that sometimes I walk with a limp. The first time I experienced this, it lasted for six months. At the beginning of this part of the journey, they gave me physical therapy for four weeks. Doctors still weren't sure what was causing the ataxia, and they hoped that the therapy would help with my muscle memory. Tests showed that there was nothing wrong with the nerves and muscles in my legs. It was all in my brain. During an attack or episode, the part of my brain that controls muscle memory doesn't work correctly. When I am walking with a limp, the other parts of my leg and hip are not moving correctly either. This can lead to hip pain and even a fall. During physical therapy, I learned how my leg and foot are supposed to move when I walk. I never had to focus on thinking about the movement of my leg and foot before. I gained an understanding of how these parts of my body work together to allow me to walk correctly. During this time, they gave me a cane. The cane provided stability while I focused on the coordination of my leg movement.

I learned that the ability to walk depends heavily on what is happening in my brain. Because of my disorder, there is nothing the doctors can do to fix what is going on in my brain. The support I have to help me walk correctly is a cane. In the beginning, I was not appreciative of having to use a cane. I really struggled with it. People could see that I had a problem, and that was the biggest issue for me. I remember walking to the entrance of a store at the same time as an elderly-looking person. We would both stop at the door and wait for the other to enter. I remember thinking, *Why is this person waiting for me? Clearly, as a younger person, I should let them go first.* Then I would realize that they were letting me go first because I was walking with a cane. Sometimes, I felt like a disabled person on the cane because I thought that's how others saw me. The lack of coordination in my leg was in my brain. The problem I had with walking with a cane was in my mind. I was more concerned about what people thought than living my best life. Naturally, people are concerned when they see you walking with a cane, especially when you don't normally do so. I would always say that I didn't want people to feel sorry for me, but I can't control how others feel. I can only control what I think and how I react and feel.

When I am experiencing ataxia, the cane is a blessing. If I didn't have the cane, I wouldn't be able to get around safely. At least once or twice each year, I have to use my cane for at least a week at a time. I'm thankful that I have this tool. It allows me to continue to take part in my daily activities despite my condition. It allows me to keep my independence because my family knows that I can get around safely. I have accepted that this condition is a part of my life indefinitely, so when I experience the weakness that I know comes with this condition, I just grab my support.

When God tells Paul that His strength is perfect in weakness, He is letting Paul know that in the insufficiency of his natural condition, God is his strength. God knows we are not sufficient in ourselves. Our strength must come from Him. As much as we can do on our own, we can never accomplish our Kingdom purpose if we don't rely on God's strength. When we experience weakness, there can be a tendency to become discouraged and even give up. This is not how God sees our weakness. God has always known our natural limitations. In fact, the biggest roadblock we have is how we think about our own abilities. When we don't recognize weakness within ourselves, we gain a false sense of self-confidence. We can be in danger of thinking that we are enough and even have pride in our own abilities. We never want to be seen as weak among men, so we suffer from the spirit of competition and neglect to work in the spirit of cooperation. We want to do it on our own. The problem with this is if I do it on my own, then I get all the credit. When does God get the glory? The greatest accomplishment I can have is for God to get the glory out of my life. We want to see a miracle, but are we ready to be the miracle?

When we read the Bible, we see many miracles that Jesus performed. Many of these miracles involved healing. We call them miracles because man cannot do these things. For God, it is easy to heal people. Whatever He speaks happens. Because we see so many examples of God's healing power, we know we can go to God and ask Him for healing when we are in need. Sometimes, in our pursuit of healing, we don't always see the opportunity of weakness. One example that comes to mind is that of the woman with the issue of blood. If you have read the story, you know she suffered from this illness for twelve years. She spent all her money on doctors and had been quarantined. When she heard Jesus was in town, she pressed her way to Him and received her healing. The Bible tells us she decided that if she could touch the hem of Jesus' garment, she would be made whole. She allowed that faith to turn into action, and Jesus let her know that her faith in action resulted in her healing. It was a miracle because in twelve years, no doctor had been able to do what Jesus did in a moment. If we look at this woman, we can learn some other things about her. She had perseverance. She didn't stop after one doctor couldn't heal her. Her healing was so important to her she kept seeking help even when it cost her all her money. She did not allow societal rules to stop her, either. Knowing that she was not supposed to be around people, she pushed through a crowd of people to get her healing. When she received her healing, Jesus told her that her faith had made her whole. At the moment that she touched him, He told his disciples that virtue had gone out of him. I learned that when we touch God in accordance with His will, He responds. If you look at that story of this woman, you see she had the character needed to put herself in position to activate the spirit of God in her life. Though she is an example of faith in action, she shows much more. It is her faith that motivated her to keep moving even when it took twelve years, spending all her money and disobeying societal norms. God sustained her for all those years. Somehow, she made it one day at a time until she could get to Jesus. Nothing in the Bible said that she had a bunch of help and support from people. We can even assume that she was poor because she spent all her money on doctors. What kept her going through all of this?

There are things we are going to have to suffer in this life to build up our godly character. If this woman had never suffered from that condition, she may never have seen the need to push so hard to get to Jesus. To her, getting to Jesus was worth whatever it may have cost her to be out in public with her condition. I believe that God still wants us to be just as desperate to get to Him for everything. When we get desperate for God, we depend on Him for our very life. One line from a song says, "You are the air I breathe." This shows that I cannot do anything without God. Often, it is our weakness that will help us get to this place.

I struggled with my cane because it showed what I struggle with most days. Without the cane, no one can see the aches and the pain. No one can see the physical and mental exhaustion that has become a reality in my life. While the cane provides support when my legs are not working correctly, I go to God daily for strength to get out of bed and perform daily tasks. The experience that I have with physical weakness has become an opportunity for me to gain spiritual strength. Even in my mind, I wonder how I will make it through the hard days. My faith in God keeps me pressing so that I can live in the will of God. I found the path of walking in the spirit through weakness. Over time, I've learned that the daily prayer for strength has to go beyond the strength I need to perform natural tasks. I remember God has called me to fulfill His purpose. This weakness is present to perfect His power in me. It allows me to draw from God's strength. I need God's strength to do something that I could never do on my own. The battle is seeing weakness the way God sees it. Therefore, our mindset has to change. I had been afraid to display this weakness because I saw it as an indication of what I could no longer do. As I work to see things God's way, I see this weakness as an opportunity to pursue God's will in my life. My cane has become a symbol of freedom and power. I am not looking to gain physical strength. I am looking for and expecting the power of God to take over so that I can accomplish that to which He has called me. There is so much more in me that God wants to use. I want God to use me completely for His purpose and for His glory. The only limitations I truly have are those that I put on myself. Sometimes I view life through my natural limitations. In those times, the battle is truly in my mind. The enemy will bring negative thoughts to my mind to discourage me from pursuing my purpose. I've learned that God will provide a vision, but it is up to us to put the work in making the vision operational. God has given us that power and responsibility. That's why James says that faith without works is dead. It doesn't matter how much I say I believe in God if I won't take the action needed to make it happen. When we truly walk by faith, God makes the provision. Sometimes we let fear stop us from acting. It is in that fear that the enemy works fiercely to keep us from moving forward. For me, it was worrying about how others would see me and not give me an opportunity. This is truly what some call "stinkin' thinkin'." I was giving power to others instead of looking to God. If God is truly in control of our lives, we must learn to look to Him for everything. If God has called me to do something, I have to trust that He will provide everything I need to accomplish it. He just wants me to have enough faith in Him to keep pursuing His purpose no matter what happens in this life. God is never caught off guard. When He created me, He knew every challenge that I would face. The truth is that He knew that these challenges would be opportunities for me if I would give myself to Him.

Chapter Eight

IT'S A CHRONIC DISORDER

I've been wearing eyeglasses since I was six years old. I was diagnosed with myopia, more commonly known as nearsightedness. There is no cure for myopia, and over time, my condition has gotten worse. By the time I reached my forties, I found I struggled to read small print that was close in proximity. Fortunately, I go to the optometrist each year to get my eyes examined, and they prescribe corrective lenses that address both disorders. Wearing glasses helps me to live a normal life. I can read, drive, and get around safely because of a medical intervention we all know as corrective lenses. I do not write this with sarcasm, but I am making a point. When I researched the definition of chronic disorders or diseases, I found that in the medical world it is broadly defined as "conditions that last 1 year or more and require ongoing medical attention or limit activities of daily living or both" (Centers for Disease Control, 2021). Using that definition, I could categorize my nearsightedness as a chronic disorder. Medical science calls it an error or a focus disorder. Nevertheless, I choose to use this example to help me find my new normal as I embrace the conditions with which I now live.

The doctors diagnosed me with protein S deficiency and hemiplegic migraine. Not only are these disorders chronic, but they are also rare. Protein S deficiency is a disorder that causes abnormal blood clotting.

Hemiplegic migraine is a rare type of migraine with aura that occurs with motor weakness during the aura.

Based upon what I have been told and have researched, I understand I was born with both conditions. Without genetic testing, one will not know that they have these conditions until they experience symptoms. In my case, I developed deep vein thrombosis and then pulmonary embolisms twice. You can't tell that I have protein S deficiency by looking at me. I will take an anticoagulant every day for the rest of my life. When I was first prescribed the medication, I asked the nurse if I didn't have to worry about getting a blood clot since I was on the medication, and she told me no. This was absolutely true because during my first pregnancy, I developed pulmonary embolisms while on an anticoagulant. At that time, I had not been diagnosed with the clotting disorder, so they were giving me the medication as a precaution. This incident led to the diagnosis.

I live with this disorder by taking my medication, watching what I eat (some foods counteract the effectiveness of the medication), and making life adjustments. For example, when I travel, if we are driving, I have to make sure that I stop and walk around every two and a half to three hours. I have to have my INR checked regularly to make sure that my blood stays in the therapeutic range. That means that I walk around every day as someone whose blood is in a "less coagulated" state. This puts me at risk of internal bleeding every day. If I fall, I have to go to the emergency room to make sure there is no internal bleeding. As a result, I limit activities that could cause a fall as much as I can. No one wants to fall on purpose, so limiting such activities may seem simple. For me, this means I have to take the time to weigh the risk of falling on activities for which I may never have in the past. I can no longer ride a bicycle. At my age, it may not seem important, but I definitely think about it as my kids grow up and become more independent on their bicycles. Walking to the car in the wintertime can be a significant challenge since falling on the ice will result in a trip to the hospital. Once, my dog was trying to run out of the kitchen door. I fell and hit my head as I tried to go after her. We spent the next few hours in the ER, ensuring that I did not have internal bleeding. I was even in a terrible car accident, and my car was totaled. Thankfully, in these cases, God protected me, and I did not experience the bleeding.

To make matters more interesting, I once fell outside after a winter storm. It was more of a slow descent to the ground. I knew I would be sore, but I didn't fall hard, so I just expected the soreness. By the end of the night, I could barely walk to my bedroom. I realized that even though I did not experience internal bleeding and bruising from the fall, the experience triggered my other disorder, hemiplegic migraine.

The effects of having protein S deficiency are potentially life-threatening. Having hemiplegic migraine, though not life-threatening, can be more debilitating. When triggered, I can lose the ability to speak, walk, or move my arms. Sometimes my speech slows and includes stuttering. Sometimes I experience an ataxic gait, so I cannot control my leg when I walk. This results in me walking with a limp, and I need a cane so that I don't fall because of the lack of coordination. When I fell after the storm, I was on my cane for a month.

There are many challenges to living with chronic disorders. The first is trying to adjust to the fact that there is no cure for these conditions and understanding that you have to make changes so that you can live a full life in your new normal. To me, this has been the hardest part of my journey. For the first few years, I treated my conditions like a sickness. I thought I could take my meds and work to overcome these disorders. I thought that success was being able to do all the things I used to do the way I used to do them. As I write this, I don't remember the last time I felt normal. I don't remember what it feels like to get up in the morning and feel refreshed from a full night's sleep. I used to rely on my memory heavily. I could process many things in my mind and remember what I needed to do. Now, I rely on lists and patterns of behavior. Sometimes, I can't remember the words to songs or how to play songs on the piano I have played for years. It's not that the information isn't there; it's just hard for me to access it in my brain. I have always been a thinker. I enjoy the process of problem-solving, but in my new normal, this has become a struggle. It is most difficult when I am tired. Did I mention that chronic fatigue is a part of my new normal? Sometimes I feel like I am trapped in my body and in my brain, knowing what I want to do but not being able to make it happen. I spent eleven years of my life trying not to lose myself. I fought to be who I was before the conditions. I didn't want to live a life of limitations. I didn't want people to feel sorry for me and think I couldn't do anything because I was "sick." The only thing I could see was what I was losing. I think that is an interesting part of the grief that comes with loss. I had spent so much time thinking about what I was losing that I never considered what I might be gaining. In my fight, I prayed for God to heal me, and I believed that He would. I am a two-time survivor of pulmonary embolism in both lungs. I know God has His hands on me. I know that He still has work for me to do or He would have taken me years ago. Sometimes, when we pray, we just expect God to do what we ask Him to do. There are Scriptures that support that in the context of God's will for us. At one point, I came to realize that God would not heal me from these conditions. Since I accepted God's will for me, I have begun the journey to victory. In order for me to accept God's will, I had to give up my own. I had to give up my idea about what normal is and pursue the new normal that God had ordained for me. God knew these disorders were in my body from the time I was born. He kept me and didn't let them stop me from accomplishing my assignment. Usually, people with clotting disorders have miscarriages. I have had two pregnancies, and by the grace of God, I have delivered two healthy girls. People die from one blood clot in the lung. I am still alive, having experienced multiple blood clots in both lungs. There are people with hemiplegic migraine who cannot work or drive. As I write this, I can still do both. I am extremely blessed and thankful.

I now refer to myself as someone who lives with chronic disorders. As long as God gives me breath in my body, I know that He still has a plan for me, and I am committed to doing His will. I have learned to stop focusing on my limitations and to seek God for what and how. I am no longer fighting to live like I don't have these disorders. I have embraced them. I am no longer asking God to heal me. I am asking Him to show me what He wants me to do each day, and I am trusting Him to supply whatever I need to do it.

Chapter Nine

SUPERHEROES: FINDING AND EMBRACING MY IDENTITY

My favorite type of movie is action-adventure movies with storylines involving superheroes. I don't know why, but I really enjoy watching the story unfold as these enhanced people use their powers for the good of humanity. In the modern version of these types of movies, the superhero is more relatable because they also struggle with real-life issues. Batman struggles with the loss of his parents through violent crime. Thor has serious issues with relationships, as he has grown up with a dysfunctional family. Even Captain America, in all his wholesomeness, struggles with loneliness. Their powers are gifts to the world, and as they can conquer physical threats, they are constantly battling human issues within themselves. In the end, they may conquer the bad guy or girl, but they are always in search of solutions for their own struggle. This is their life. The message I take away from their stories is that there are some struggles in this life that are common to all human beings. Even with super intelligence, the ability to fly, and super strength, they could not escape life's struggles.

If we are not careful, we can fall into a place where we view our lives through our gifts. God has gifted each one of us. When God created us, He had a Kingdom purpose in mind and gifted us accordingly. I mention this often as I am ministering. Sometimes people will say they don't have a gift, but this is not true. The problem with society/people is that we look at the gifts that have value in this society. We categorize people who can provide entertainment or can achieve some extraordinary task as gifted, while everyone else is called ordinary. This is man's view, but it is not God's view. In this context, I am speaking about the talents that God has given us. These are abilities we didn't earn. Often, you don't truly understand your gift because it's just part of who you are. It's how you think. It's how God made you. There are gifted writers, teachers, caregivers, singers, artisans, speakers, and the list goes on and on. The thing to remember is that God placed this gift in you because it is purposeful in His Kingdom.

I have learned that I am gifted in teaching. I love teaching and have been blessed to use this gift to affect many young people. It has truly amazed me when people have expressed how they enjoyed my classes or when students come back to say how much they were helped by being in my class. I've even had teachers talk about how they benefited from a professional development session that I led. The most amazing thing about all of this is that I have never felt like I had this exceptional ability as a teacher. I loved watching the "light bulb" come on for people. For me, I wanted to be an excellent teacher, and it challenged me over the years to reach my students. Many times, I would come up with ideas, and it amazed me how they worked. Sometimes people would ask me how I could get the students to perform, and I didn't understand it myself. I always put the work in, but I was always nervous about the outcome. Over the years, I have been recognized for my work in education through awards and promotions. I have been truly blessed. When I started suffering with my disorders, I struggled to work like I was used to working. Sometimes it's hard for me to focus and think because I suffer from fatigue. The lack of confidence in my ability to continue in my job was the biggest problem I had. I couldn't serve in the school setting anymore. My body did not allow me to keep up with the pace, but I still knew how to do the job. For a long time, I fought. I thought maybe I could find a position that would allow me to keep teaching and still be okay. I didn't want to face my reality because I could only see what I was losing. The problem was that I could only see the value of my gift in the context of working in a school system. When I could no longer keep up that pace, I felt like I was failing. I felt like my only choice was to give up my profession and retire on disability. I even requested the paperwork so I could begin the process. I met with a representative, and he explained I could no longer teach or write curriculum if I retired on disability. Those words haunted me. I knew I could not keep up with the pace of working in a traditional educational setting, but in my heart, I knew that there was more for me to do. There were dreams I had pushed to the side that would require me to teach as I waited for retirement. I even used this gift in the church, but I hadn't considered using it for the Kingdom. People let me know they benefited from my ministry. By this time, I understood God had given me a gift to reach people in this way.

The interesting thing about being in trouble is that it is the time we become most diligent in seeking God. It is in the time of weakness that we acknowledge our limitations and look to God for guidance and strength. At least this happens to me. As I struggled to face the reality of chronic illness daily, I found it difficult to carry out tasks that had come so easily to me before. This experience taught me I was relying on my strength and knowledge to accomplish these things. Where my strength and knowledge are limited is where I would have to stop. This was a frightening reality for me. I felt stuck. I was stuck in my mind. I had been living my best life, but I wasn't living an abundant life. In this space, I looked to God and said, "I need you." This statement is one that I have made before, but this time, I needed God to help me get out of bed. I needed Him all along, but I wasn't thinking that way when it didn't hurt to move. I always needed Him to help me figure out how to complete projects at work, but I wasn't desperately leaning on Him until I couldn't gather my thoughts and organize a plan. I always thanked God and gave him honor for the things I had accomplished, but I had become comfortable using the abilities He gave me. An example I can use here is David. David was a man of many gifts and talents. In his younger years, we see the gifts at work as he slays Goliath with stones and a slingshot. When David tells the king that he can slay the giant, he speaks with confidence about who God is to him. He references how he killed a lion and a bear with God, and it is with this confidence that he knows he can slay the giant. David was also a gifted musician. The king would call for David when he was troubled in his spirit, and David's playing would drive evil spirits away. While we can clearly see why the king would find use for David, we must remember that God had anointed him to the purpose of being king before these things happened to David. As David walks the path to his destiny, the king becomes jealous of him and seeks to have him killed. David runs and lives like a fugitive. Even though God put him on a path to be king, David lives like King Saul's word is greater than God's. Eventually, David comes to himself, and as he aligns his mindset with God's will, God works on his behalf. Saul accepts the fact that David is to be king.

Like David, God defines our identity from the beginning. God equips us to live out this identity here in this world. As we live this natural experience, we will have struggles. All human beings deal with natural struggles. We may not all have the same struggles, but we all have them. The challenge of overcoming is to remember who God says you are. In this life, it is so easy to get into a routine. If things are going well, we continue the routine. Life's struggles and trials help us gauge where we are in our minds. Before this illness showed up, I felt like I was doing well. To me, I had a bright future. I was at the top of my career, and there seemed to be so many possibilities for me. My view of success was defined by my status in this society. I wasn't sinning. I wasn't neglecting church and my duties there. I was excelling there too. It's so easy to get distracted by natural success. As much as I existed in this place of what I considered success, to God, I was in a place of limitation. God had so much more planned for me. As I suffered from the symptoms of my illnesses, I had time to stop and really seek God for what He wanted me to do. I learned that what I thought I had lost put me in a place of gaining with God. When I let go of the things that I thought made me successful, God opened doors to things that I never believed I could truly have. There were so many things that I wanted to do in my dreams, but with limited vision and fear of losing, I tucked them away. Every time I did not move toward the vision God had given me, I lost a part of myself. I remember having a conversation with a former supervisor about where my career seemed to be going. I was well-respected and had proved capable on the job. Inside, I felt like I was dying. I felt like I was in a box. I was in a box, but I put myself there trying to be what I thought the organization wanted me to be. I was willing to give up who I was just until I could achieve the position that I wanted. I achieved that position in another district, and I found out that it was not for me. I finally realized that the issue was not with the organizations. God had a plan for me, but I was not pursuing it. God allowed me to have these jobs as a provision. I allowed these jobs to become my identity. Who I was became defined by what I could achieve in the eyes of people, and there is no fulfillment in that. Early in my career, I attended a conference focused on education in urban settings. It was one of the best conferences I have ever attended. There, I heard national leaders in education speak, and I was truly inspired. Fast forward to my twenty-seventh year in my career, and I had the opportunity to work with one of these noted leaders as we worked to implement a new system in the district. Not only was I working with this guru in education, but I was also working to implement a system that I truly believed would benefit students. It was work that I had begun years prior, and I was now working in a district that was committed to that same work. One morning, we had a meeting with the consultant, and he even commended me on my thoughts and conclusions regarding the work. It didn't hit me until I was getting ready for bed that night that I was truly in a different place. I realized that I wasn't as excited about the work. I knew it was good work and that I had been passionate about it, but I didn't feel the same way about doing this work. I didn't even share my interactions with my mom or my husband. It was just another day at the job. That realization was a shock to me. At first, I felt sad, but then I understood that this was a good change for me. It was good work, but it was not *my* purpose. Doing good work as an educator is something I should do, but it is not who I am. It does not define me. My illness doesn't define me either. I am a vessel created by God to be used for His divine purpose. As I journey through this life, I will have many experiences. Many of these experiences have helped to mold me into who I am today. Viewing my life from this perspective has set me on a path to true freedom. My struggle with finding contentment in this new part of my life was centered in an identity crisis. I had defined myself based upon what I could accomplish specifically as an educator. I had found my niche and success in this field. This was how I saw myself, but it was not how God saw me. When God created me, he saw much more than I ever could. This is why we must learn to walk by faith. The truth is I don't know everything God has in store for me. I don't have an understanding of all that God wants to accomplish through me. I have learned that I must submit myself totally to Him. When I say that God knows what's best for me, I say it with the understanding that He can see things that I cannot. I may know how I feel, but my feelings are based on my limited knowledge and experience. When I think I can't do something, it's based upon my limitations. This is why there is such a struggle with change. Even when God is directing us to shift, we wrestle with the idea. The struggle is not because we don't love God. We don't understand the battle. We have to learn to live like we belong to God. The enemy would like for us to believe that we are what happens to us. So many times, we don't have control over what happens to us, and in those times, we feel helpless and sometimes even hopeless. The Bible tells us, "The Lord directs the steps of the godly. He delights in every detail of their lives." (Ps 37:23) This assures me that things are not just happening to me. God is intentional. He knows who He wants me to be. This experience has shaken me, but it didn't shake God. It has pushed me into a time of examination. It has given me an opportunity to truly trust God for everything. It has helped me to move out of my comfort zone and onto the path that God has set for me toward my identity.

An important lesson I have learned is that my gift is not my identity. How I use my gift is often determined by who I choose to be. For every superhero, there is a supervillain. They both have enhanced abilities. The difference is who they are as a person. Superheroes are people of character and commitment, so when they possess extraordinary skills and enhanced abilities, they use those strengths for good. When we go back to David in the Bible, we see someone who was called, not for his ability as a great warrior or his musical talent. He was chosen by God because he was a man after God's own heart.

I've learned the importance of knowing my true identity. Who has God called me to be? When I have figured out who God wants me to be, I can use my gifts and talents for His glory. I have become less concerned about my circumstances and more focused on being who God has called me to be. My focus on living out my identity has helped me to put things into perspective. Everything I have suffered has helped me to come to this reality. I am who God says I am, and that's who I am required to be.

Chapter Ten

RECEIVING GOD'S GRACE

After all this time and with everything that I have experienced, I have come to an understanding. God has allowed me to be in a position to receive His grace. I never imagined that suffering could bring me to this place. In the Bible, we have examples of miracles that God has performed. One example of suffering that is often used is that of Job. God allowed Job to suffer significant loss because God favored him. God knew Job would always be faithful to Him, no matter what happened in his life. When Satan was looking for someone to destroy, God offered him Job. That statement may sound a little strange, but that's what actually happened. God knew Job's heart, and He knew He could trust Job with this temptation. Job lost everything: his family, his wealth, and even his health. Through all of it, Job felt horrible, but he never blamed God. He never lost reverence for God. He didn't understand why he was going through such suffering, and it hurt him, but he continued to honor God as God through it all. Job's friends and family didn't encourage him. He was all alone in his situation, and yet he still proclaimed God as sovereign. I've read Job's story over the years, and I admired his commitment to God. He was truly a man of integrity.

As I studied Job, I came to realize that Job was in a place of favor. Mostly, when we think of God's favor, we are referring to receiving blessings like a promotion on the job or something like that. Job was in a place of favor from the beginning of the story. God favored him because he honored God. Like many humans, the devil saw God's favor in the things that Job had. He told God that Job only served Him because of the things he had. God knew Job's heart. He knew that Job's commitment was in his heart. So, He kept Job with a mind to continue to serve Him through all his suffering and loss. All this suffering became an opportunity for God to get the glory out of Job's life.

It is often said that it is easy to praise God when things are going well. This is an accurate statement. In those times, we speak of God's grace. Grace is having favor in God's sight. The key to grace is that we have done nothing to earn this favor. We can do nothing to deserve this favor. In order to better understand how we are favored, we must understand that God is absolute. His Word is absolute. When the Word says "the wages of sin is death," it means that because we were all born in sin, we deserve death. We do not deserve to experience life with God. Yet because of His grace, we can experience life with Him through Jesus Christ. The other part is understanding that this favor is in God's sight. As human beings, we often look at favor from the natural perspective. When things are going well in our natural lives, we speak about the favor of God. We understand that every day we get up, we are living under God's grace.

I have come to the understanding that even though God grants grace, we don't always receive His grace and live like we understand what God has given us. We are often so blinded by this natural life that we cannot always see that God has called us to live by His grace. When we live a

life that God has called us to, we are acknowledging His grace toward us.

When our lives are out of focus, we cannot please God, so He may allow

us to experience things that will help us get back to our place of purpose.

By now, you may see where I am going with this. I finally came to an

understanding about all that I have suffered in my body. These diseases

seemed to come "out of the blue." I had never really been sick before, not

even with the flu. There were people who wondered if I had been cursed

or if I had done something wrong. I knew that was not the case. When

I was in the hospital, hooked up to IVs and machines, the peace of God

sustained me. I knew that if I died, I was going to be with Jesus because of

the life I was living. The struggle was not between me and God. The actual

struggle was internal because of what people said and what I thought about

what I was suffering. I was uncomfortable with the suffering because I saw

loss from a natural perspective. It took me a long time to see God's grace

in this. His grace was there all the time. I wasn't receiving it. I thought

that favor would be Him healing me. I didn't see the opportunity for me to

honor God in this weakness. God is a patient teacher. I kept secrets about

these illnesses because I didn't want people to see me down and broken. I

had an image of what I thought I should look like, and I thought that was

what people should see. When God created me, He had an image of what I

should look like, and my image conflicted with His image. When you walk

with God, He allows you to experience things that will help transform us

into His image. Since we are born in sin, we are imperfect in His eyes. So, we need His grace. We benefit from His favor while He works on us. The Bible tells us in the twelfth chapter of Romans that we are transformed by the renewing of our minds. God is trying to change our thinking to align with His thinking. We don't see ourselves like He sees us. He sees us as victorious from a spiritual perspective. He sees us carrying out the purpose to which He has called us through obedience to Him. It takes complete obedience to God to accomplish our purpose. We are often in our own way because we keep trying to make spiritual gains through natural means. This is not how God works. In this spiritual walk, I have learned that we must give up everything to please God. We must trust God totally. To get to that place, God will allow us to lose things that were important to us in the natural world so that we may gain what we need in the spiritual world. I'll be honest. My job and professional standing were important to me. My natural abilities were important to me. Giving them up has been difficult because I saw my success through my natural abilities. I always acknowledged that God gave me these abilities. As human beings, we will do that, but that does not equate to spiritual victory.

Giving up is the actual struggle. I equated giving up with quitting or not trying. To give up is to surrender. I'm surrendering my way to follow God's way. This entails giving up my way of thinking for God's way of thinking. I can embrace all the changes that have come with having a chronic illness because I now understand that God is my source. When He created me, He knew that this would be a part of me, yet He still saw me as useful in His grand plan. My weaknesses are not a hindrance to God because He has all power. In the Old Testament, God used a donkey to speak to a prophet who was going down a wrong path. He used a burning bush to speak to Moses. He even used a rock to supply water for the children of Israel. There is a hymn that says, "Trees don't want to be mountains, they just praise the Lord." Animals, plants, and rocks have no will, so they always operate under the will of God. I don't believe that God had to have a conversation with the donkey, bush, or the rock to use them in the way that He chose to use them. As human beings, the actual struggle is to always submit ourselves to the will of God. Many times, we want God's goodness and His blessings, but we want them our way. We want to define our own success when God has called us to greater. Greater is defined by God, not humanity.

I've learned that giving up is my greatest victory. By letting go of my own ideas about what made me normal and successful, I could turn to God's idea about these things. I don't have to be everything to everybody. I just have to be available to God. Now I want to take a moment to explore this a little more deeply. I've spoken about unrealistic expectations many times. The system of this world is rooted in unrealistic expectations. No matter how hard you work, even with great intentions and a pure motive, somebody won't be satisfied. God is not like that at all. He is satisfied with our obedience to Him. In the sight of God, kindness to a stranger on the street is just as great as preaching His Word to a stadium full of people. I finally understood that obedience to God is easier than pleasing people. The real battle was in my mind. If God is pleased with me, it doesn't matter what is happening in my body, nor does it matter what others may think about me. God was using chronic illness to help me get to my real potential. When I stopped fighting, trying to be who I was, I turned to God to learn who He wanted me to be. Every time I gave up something I could no longer do, I could see something else God wanted me to do. I started doing things that were in my heart to do and that I could never do before.

Often, I've asked God to do so many things for me. I've learned on this journey that God has equipped me to do everything He has called me to do. He has been waiting for me to get to work. Sometimes in my life, I have been disgruntled because I've worked so hard, and I felt like people didn't appreciate me or even took advantage of me. This was definitely the case when I started experiencing the symptoms associated with my illnesses. I thought I had earned a place of respect based on the work I had done. I was devastated when I learned that was not the case. I had to learn that it wasn't personal. It's the way of this world. Then I thought about it from God's perspective. Here, God created me with gifts and talents, and I focused my energies on how everyone else received what I had to give. I allowed myself to believe that my worth was determined by their acceptance of me. I didn't truly understand that what I have is precious because God said so. I owe God my very life, and that means I must use whatever I have for His glory.

I understand that my weakness has freed me. I no longer have to depend on my strength. God is more than enough for me. Being who He created me to be is satisfying to me. I am enough because of who He is. I no longer feel the need to hide my weakness from anyone. It is a part of my humanity, but it does not determine my destiny. Chronic illness was once a disruption in my life. Thankfully, I now see it as an opportunity. It was an opportunity for me to reflect upon who I really was and who God wants me to be. The Bible lets us know God cannot lie. He is not capable of lying. He is, and His Word is. This means that whatever God has said about us is completely true. No circumstance can negate God's Word. When we choose to walk by faith, we are choosing to believe what God has said about us and continue in His path, no matter what happens. This journey has given me the opportunity to grow closer to God. I learned to lean on Him for everything. As I grew closer to Him, I could hear His voice more clearly. What God said to me and about me is more profound than anything that may happen to me. God told the prophet Jeremiah, "Before you were formed in your mother's womb, I knew you" (Jer 1:5). The same is true for you and me. God knew who He wanted me to be. My job is to walk in agreement with what God has spoken. In embracing my weakness, my strength comes from God, and my ability to be all that He has called me to be is through Him. God has used chronic illness to perfect His power in me. He has taught me how to draw my strength from Him. Those things that I thought were limiting are now empowering. I no longer feel the need to hide these things that were once seen as weaknesses. They will not stop me from accomplishing my God-given purpose.

The Bible tells us to rejoice in tribulation. We often rejoice after the tribulation. We rejoice because God spared our lives, and that is in order, but rejoicing in tribulation takes another level of faith. Even if the situation doesn't change, we still rejoice. These situations will help us understand where we are in our faith walk. As we learn to go through these tribulations without losing our faith in God, we gain more patience, experience, and hope. I was born with chronic illness, and God knew when the symptoms would bring me closer to Him. I can rejoice because God loves me so much that He held back the symptoms until I could benefit from this experience.

". . . Now I take limitations in stride, and with good cheer, these limitations that cut me down to size-abuse, accidents, opposition, bad breaks. I just let Christ take over! And so the weaker I get, the stronger I become." (2 Cor 12:10 MSG)

REFERENCES

About chronic diseases. (2022, July 21). CDC. https://www.cdc.gov/ chronicdisease/about/index.htm

Dictionary by Merriam-Webster: America's most-trusted online dictionary. (n.d.). Merriam-Webster. Retrieved July 25, 2022, from http://merriam-webster.com

Familiar or sporadic hemiplegic migraine - About the Disease. (n.d.). Genetic and Rare Diseases Information Center. Retrieved July 25, 2022, from https://rarediseases.info.nih.gov/diseases/10768/familiar-or-sporadic-hemiplegic-migraine.

Protein S deficiency - About the Disease. (n.d.). Genetic and Rare Diseases Information Center. Retrieved July 25, 2022, from https://rarediseases.info.nih.gov/diseases/4524/protein-s-deficiency.